Natural Hormone Balance for Women

A Holistic Guide to Restoring Hormonal Balance and Enhancing Women's Wellness

Graham Julian Oliver

Disclaimer

The information provided in *Natural Hormone Balance for Women: A Holistic Guide to Restoring Hormonal Balance and Enhancing Women's Wellness* is intended solely for educational and informational purposes. This book does not constitute medical, health, or professional advice and should not be used as a substitute for consultation with qualified healthcare providers. Always seek the guidance of your physician or other qualified health professionals with any questions you may have regarding your health or medical condition. The use of any information in this book is solely at your own risk.

The author and publisher disclaim any liability arising from the use or application of the contents of this book, including any harm, side effects, or other health-related outcomes. The information provided in this book is based on the author's research, experiences, and knowledge available at the time of writing. However, the science of health and wellness is constantly evolving, and the information in this book may not reflect the most current research.

The author does not endorse or recommend any specific individual, product, website, organization, or entity mentioned in this book. Any references to third-party products, brands, services, websites, or other entities are solely for informational purposes and do not imply any endorsement, recommendation, affiliation, or approval. Readers are encouraged to perform their own research and consult healthcare professionals before relying on any information provided herein.

By reading this book, you acknowledge and agree to these terms.

About This Book

"Natural Hormone Balance for Women: A Holistic Guide to Restoring Hormonal Balance and Enhancing Women's Wellness" serves as an essential resource for women seeking to understand and improve their hormonal health. In a world where hormonal imbalances can affect everything from mood and energy levels to reproductive health, this guide emphasizes the importance of recognizing and addressing these issues holistically. By considering not just the physical aspects of health but also emotional and lifestyle factors, women can cultivate a more profound understanding of how to restore balance and enhance their overall wellness.

At the heart of this book lies the exploration of hormones and their critical roles in various bodily functions. Hormones regulate mood, metabolism, and reproductive health; however, imbalances can lead to significant health challenges, including fatigue, anxiety, and menstrual irregularities. By understanding the intricate dance of hormones like estrogen, progesterone, and cortisol, women can identify the signs of imbalance and take proactive steps toward restoration. The discussion extends to factors that influence hormonal health, including diet, stress, and environmental elements, and sheds light on the importance of hormone testing as a vital tool for managing health.

The book's holistic approach emphasizes the necessity of addressing root causes rather than merely alleviating symptoms. Nutrition plays a pivotal role in hormonal balance, and the book provides insights into foods that support hormone production while highlighting those that should be avoided. From the impact of nutrient deficiencies to the benefits of a Mediterranean diet, readers are equipped with practical advice on meal planning and the significance of meal timing. The connection between hydration and hormone regulation is also explored, offering a comprehensive view of how nutrition can be a powerful ally in achieving hormonal harmony.

Stress management emerges as another crucial theme in maintaining hormonal health. The guide delves into the connection between stress and hormone levels, providing effective techniques for stress reduction, including mindfulness practices, exercise, and sleep hygiene. By creating a balanced routine that prioritizes relaxation and social support, women can build resilience against the daily pressures that disrupt hormonal equilibrium. The book further discusses the benefits of physical activity, detailing how various forms of exercise impact hormone levels, emphasizing the importance of regular movement, rest, and finding enjoyable activities to stay motivated.

Natural remedies also play a significant role in the quest for hormonal balance, and the guide offers an overview of herbal supplements, essential oils, and traditional therapies. It stresses the importance of consulting healthcare professionals to ensure safety and efficacy while exploring the research behind these natural treatments. This holistic perspective acknowledges the value of combining natural remedies with conventional medicine for a well-rounded approach to health.

The impact of hormonal imbalances on women's lives cannot be overstated, as the book outlines common conditions such as PCOS and menopause, exploring their symptoms and implications. It highlights the critical link between hormonal health and mental well-being, addressing how imbalances can affect weight, metabolism, and sleep patterns. By encouraging women to advocate for their health and seek medical advice when necessary, the book empowers readers to take control of their hormonal health journey.

Additionally, the guide examines environmental factors that can disrupt hormonal balance, such as endocrine disruptors and toxins. It provides actionable strategies for reducing exposure to harmful substances, promoting sustainable living practices that protect hormonal health. By fostering awareness about personal care products and environmental health risks, the book equips women with the knowledge needed to create safer living spaces.

Maintaining hormonal balance over time is a lifelong commitment, and the book emphasizes the importance of regular monitoring and building a supportive healthcare team. By adapting lifestyle changes as they age and celebrating small victories along the way, women can cultivate resilience against hormonal fluctuations. The resource also encourages open discussions about hormonal health and emphasizes the significance of self-compassion in the process of achieving and maintaining balance.

With common concerns and FAQs addressed throughout the book, readers gain practical insights into recognizing signs of hormonal imbalance and tracking their health. This guide not only provides a wealth of information but also fosters a sense of community and support among women seeking to enhance their wellness. Through a comprehensive understanding of hormonal health and a commitment to holistic practices, "Natural Hormone Balance for Women" empowers women to reclaim their well-being and thrive.

Table of Contents

Introduction

Understanding Hormones and Their Role

Hormones are chemical messengers that regulate numerous body functions, including mood, metabolism, immune response, and reproductive health. They are produced by various glands and work in harmony to maintain homeostasis, ensuring that your body operates efficiently. For instance, estrogen and progesterone are essential for the menstrual cycle and reproductive health, while thyroid hormones influence metabolism and energy levels.

To achieve optimal hormonal balance, it's essential to understand how different hormones interact within your body. Regular health check-ups can help identify hormonal imbalances through blood tests that measure hormone levels. Monitoring your body's response to stress, sleep, diet, and physical activity will also provide valuable insights into your hormonal health.

Recognizing Hormonal Imbalances

Hormonal imbalances can manifest in various ways, such as unexplained fatigue, weight gain, mood swings, anxiety, irregular menstrual cycles, and sleep disturbances. Recognizing these signs is the first step towards restoring balance. Keeping a journal of your symptoms, menstrual cycle, and lifestyle factors can help pinpoint patterns that may indicate hormonal issues.

Consulting with a healthcare provider is crucial for accurate diagnosis and treatment. They may recommend blood tests or hormonal assessments to identify specific imbalances. Additionally, consider tracking your diet, exercise, and sleep habits, as these factors can significantly influence hormonal health.

Diet and Nutrition for Hormonal Balance

A well-balanced diet rich in whole foods can play a vital role in restoring hormonal balance. Focus on incorporating plenty of fruits, vegetables, whole grains, healthy fats, and lean proteins into your meals. Foods high in fiber, such as legumes and whole grains, help regulate blood sugar levels and support healthy digestion, which is essential for hormonal health.

In addition to whole foods, consider including specific nutrients known to support hormonal balance. Omega-3 fatty acids, found in fish and flaxseeds, can help reduce inflammation, while foods rich in antioxidants, such as berries and leafy greens, can combat oxidative stress. Staying hydrated and limiting processed foods, sugar, and caffeine will further enhance your overall well-being.

Herbal Remedies for Hormonal Balance

Herbal remedies can offer natural support for hormonal balance. Herbs like chaste tree (Vitex) can help regulate menstrual cycles and alleviate PMS symptoms, while maca root is known for enhancing energy and mood. Additionally, adaptogenic herbs like ashwagandha and rhodiola can help the body adapt to stress, indirectly supporting hormonal balance.

Before starting any herbal supplement, it's essential to consult with a healthcare provider to ensure safety and efficacy. They can recommend appropriate dosages and combinations tailored to your specific hormonal needs. Incorporating herbal teas into your daily routine can also be a soothing way to promote balance and relaxation.

Lifestyle Changes for Hormonal Health

Implementing lifestyle changes can significantly improve hormonal balance. Regular exercise, such as aerobic activities, strength training, and yoga, can help reduce stress, regulate metabolism, and support overall health. Aim for at least 30 minutes of moderate exercise most days of the week to promote hormonal stability and enhance mood.

Additionally, prioritize sleep hygiene by establishing a consistent sleep schedule, creating a relaxing bedtime routine, and minimizing screen time before bed. Quality sleep is essential for hormone production and regulation, as many hormones, including cortisol and melatonin, are closely linked to sleep patterns. By adopting these lifestyle changes, you can create a supportive environment for hormonal balance.

Stress Management Techniques

Stress is a significant contributor to hormonal imbalances, as it can lead to elevated cortisol levels, which disrupt other hormones. To manage stress effectively, incorporate relaxation techniques into your daily routine. Practices such as mindfulness meditation, deep breathing exercises, and progressive muscle relaxation can help reduce stress and improve overall well-being.

Engaging in hobbies, spending time in nature, and practicing gratitude can also enhance your emotional resilience. Establishing a strong support network of friends and family allows for shared experiences and emotional support, which can be beneficial in managing stress and fostering a sense of community.

Physical Activity and Hormonal Balance

Regular physical activity is crucial for maintaining hormonal balance. Engaging in aerobic exercises, such as walking, running, or cycling, can help regulate insulin and cortisol levels, while strength training supports muscle mass and metabolism. Aim for a combination of aerobic and strength-training exercises at least three to five times a week to achieve the best results.

Incorporating activities like yoga or Pilates can also promote hormonal health by reducing stress and enhancing flexibility. These practices encourage mindfulness and body awareness, which can be beneficial in understanding how your body responds to exercise and overall well-being.

Sleep and Hormonal Health

Quality sleep is essential for maintaining hormonal balance, as many hormones are produced during sleep cycles. Aim for 7-9 hours of uninterrupted sleep each night by establishing a calming bedtime routine. This could include activities such as reading, taking a warm bath, or practicing relaxation techniques.

Create an optimal sleep environment by ensuring your bedroom is dark, cool, and quiet. Limiting caffeine intake, especially in the afternoon and evening, and avoiding screens before bedtime can also promote better sleep quality, supporting your body's natural hormonal rhythms.

The Role of Gut Health

Gut health plays a crucial role in hormonal balance, as a healthy gut microbiome can influence hormone metabolism and production. Incorporating fermented foods, such as yogurt, kefir, sauerkraut, and kimchi, into your diet can promote a healthy gut microbiome. Additionally, prebiotic-rich foods, like garlic, onions, and bananas, can help nourish beneficial gut bacteria.

To support gut health further, stay hydrated and consider a diet high in fiber. Fiber-rich foods, including whole grains, legumes, fruits, and vegetables, promote regular digestion and help maintain a healthy balance of gut bacteria, indirectly supporting hormonal health.

Hormonal Balance and Age

Hormonal changes are a natural part of aging, particularly during perimenopause and menopause when estrogen and progesterone levels fluctuate. To navigate these changes, focus on maintaining a balanced diet and regular exercise routine. Incorporating strength training can help combat muscle loss and support bone health during these transitions.

Additionally, consider natural supplements or lifestyle modifications to alleviate common symptoms associated with hormonal changes, such as hot flashes and mood swings. Consulting with a healthcare provider can provide tailored guidance to help manage these changes effectively and promote overall well-being during the aging process.

Importance of Regular Check-Ups

Regular health check-ups are essential for monitoring hormonal health and identifying potential imbalances early. Schedule annual appointments with your healthcare provider for routine screenings, blood tests, and discussions about any symptoms you may be experiencing. Being proactive about your health can help catch imbalances before they lead to more significant issues.

In addition to routine visits, stay informed about your body and hormonal health. Engage in open conversations with your healthcare provider about any concerns or changes you notice, ensuring that your care is personalized and responsive to your unique needs. By prioritizing regular check-ups, you can take charge of your hormonal health and overall wellness.

The Importance of a Holistic Approach

A Holistic Approach to Hormonal Health

A holistic approach to hormonal health involves evaluating the interplay between physical, emotional, and lifestyle factors that can affect hormone balance. Start by assessing your daily habits, such as diet, exercise, sleep, and stress management. Keeping a journal can help identify patterns and triggers related to hormonal fluctuations, allowing for more informed decisions regarding lifestyle adjustments.

Incorporating practices such as mindfulness, yoga, or meditation can significantly enhance emotional well-being, which directly impacts hormonal balance. Consider scheduling regular check-ins with a healthcare professional who specializes in holistic health to discuss your findings and develop a personalized plan that addresses your unique needs and circumstances.

Addressing Root Causes for Lasting Wellness

Instead of merely masking symptoms with medication, focus on uncovering and addressing the root causes of hormonal imbalances. This can involve evaluating your diet for processed foods, added sugars, and unhealthy fats, and replacing them with whole foods rich in nutrients. Include foods high in omega-3 fatty acids, fiber, and antioxidants, which support hormonal function and overall health.

In addition, it's essential to monitor and manage stress levels, as chronic stress can lead to hormonal disruptions. Techniques such as deep breathing exercises, regular physical activity, and time spent in nature can be effective in reducing stress. Understanding these root causes will empower you to make meaningful changes that promote long-term hormonal balance and overall wellness.

Nutrition for Hormonal Balance

Proper nutrition plays a pivotal role in restoring hormonal balance. Focus on consuming a diet rich in whole, unprocessed foods, including fruits, vegetables, lean proteins, healthy fats, and whole grains. Incorporate foods known to support hormonal health, such as leafy greens, berries, nuts, seeds, and fatty fish. Meal planning can be an effective way to ensure you have access to these foods regularly.

Additionally, consider adopting a balanced eating schedule that includes smaller, more frequent meals throughout the day to stabilize blood sugar levels and minimize insulin spikes. Staying hydrated is equally important; aim for at least eight glasses of water daily. Keeping a food diary can help you track your intake and identify any foods that may negatively impact your hormonal balance.

Exercise and Its Impact on Hormones

Regular physical activity is crucial for maintaining hormonal balance and overall health. Aim for a mix of aerobic, strength, and flexibility exercises. Incorporating at least 150 minutes of moderate-intensity exercise each week can help manage weight, reduce stress, and improve mood, all of which positively influence hormonal health.

Choose activities that you enjoy to make exercise a consistent part of your routine. Whether it's dancing, swimming, cycling, or yoga, finding something you love will make it easier to stick with. Always listen to your body; ensure you incorporate rest and recovery days to prevent burnout and overtraining, which can lead to hormonal disruptions.

Sleep Hygiene for Hormonal Balance

Quality sleep is fundamental for hormonal balance and overall wellness. Establish a consistent sleep schedule by going to bed and waking up at the same time every day, even on weekends. Create a calming bedtime routine that includes activities like reading, gentle stretching, or meditation to signal to your body that it's time to wind down.

Limit exposure to screens and bright lights at least an hour before bedtime, as these can interfere with the production of melatonin, a hormone essential for sleep. Aim for 7-9 hours of restorative sleep each night. Consider creating a sleep-friendly environment by keeping your bedroom dark, cool, and quiet to enhance your sleep quality.

Stress Management Techniques

Managing stress effectively is key to achieving hormonal balance. Identify your primary stressors and develop coping strategies tailored to your lifestyle. Techniques such as deep breathing, progressive muscle relaxation, or journaling can help alleviate immediate stress and promote emotional well-being.

Incorporate regular practices into your daily routine that foster relaxation and resilience, such as mindfulness meditation, yoga, or nature walks. Finding time for hobbies or activities that bring you joy can also be beneficial. By prioritizing stress management, you'll create a supportive environment for hormonal balance and overall health.

Herbal Remedies and Supplements

Integrating herbal remedies and supplements into your routine can provide additional support for hormonal balance. Consider consulting with a healthcare professional to determine which supplements may benefit your specific needs, such as adaptogens like ashwagandha or maca root, which may help manage stress and support hormonal health.

In addition, herbal teas such as spearmint or chasteberry may help alleviate symptoms of hormonal imbalance. When starting any new supplement or herbal remedy, begin with small doses to assess your body's response, and monitor any changes in symptoms. Keep an open line of communication with your healthcare provider throughout this process.

The Importance of Hydration

Staying adequately hydrated is essential for hormonal balance and overall health. Water supports various bodily functions, including digestion, nutrient absorption, and hormone transportation. Aim to drink at least half your body weight in ounces of water daily, and adjust based on activity level and climate.

Incorporate hydrating foods into your diet, such as fruits and vegetables, which can contribute to your daily water intake. Keep a reusable water bottle handy to remind yourself to drink throughout the day, and set hydration goals to stay accountable. Proper hydration can improve energy levels and support optimal hormonal function.

Mindfulness and Meditation Practices

Mindfulness and meditation are effective tools for enhancing emotional well-being and promoting hormonal balance. Start with just a few minutes of meditation daily, focusing on your breath and allowing your thoughts to come and go without judgment. This practice can help reduce stress and anxiety, creating a more conducive environment for hormonal stability.

Consider incorporating mindfulness into your daily activities by paying attention to the present moment, whether eating, walking, or engaging in conversations. Over time, these practices can foster a deeper connection with your body and its needs, ultimately contributing to a more balanced hormonal state.

Support Systems and Community

Building a support system is crucial for maintaining hormonal balance and overall wellness. Surround yourself with friends, family, or community groups that understand your journey and can provide encouragement and accountability. Sharing experiences and advice can create a sense of belonging and reduce feelings of isolation.

Consider seeking out support groups or online forums focused on women's health and hormonal balance. Engaging with others who share similar experiences can provide valuable insights and foster a sense of community. Don't hesitate to reach out for help when needed, whether through professional counseling or peer support.

Professional Guidance and Assessment

Consulting with a healthcare professional who specializes in women's health can provide tailored guidance and assessments for hormonal balance. Consider seeking out practitioners who use a holistic approach and can evaluate your overall health, including lifestyle, nutrition, and emotional well-being.

Regular check-ups and hormone level testing can help identify imbalances and track your progress over time. Collaborating with a professional can empower you to make informed decisions about your health, ensuring that your approach to hormonal balance is effective and sustainable.

CHAPTER 1:

The Basics of Hormones

Definition of Hormones and Their Functions

Hormones are chemical messengers produced by glands in the endocrine system that travel through the bloodstream to various tissues and organs, regulating a multitude of bodily functions. They play crucial roles in growth, metabolism, mood, reproductive processes, and overall health. By coordinating complex biological processes, hormones help maintain homeostasis and influence how the body responds to various stimuli.

Understanding hormones is essential for recognizing their impact on women's health. For instance, imbalances can lead to a range of health issues, including mood disorders, reproductive challenges, and metabolic disturbances. Gaining insights into these chemical messengers enables individuals to take proactive steps toward achieving hormonal balance.

Overview of Key Hormones in Women's Health

Several key hormones are vital for women's health, including estrogen, progesterone, and cortisol. Estrogen regulates the menstrual cycle and is crucial for reproductive health, while progesterone supports pregnancy and prepares the uterus for implantation. Cortisol, often referred to as the stress hormone, plays a role in the body's response to stress and helps regulate metabolism and immune function.

Each of these hormones must be in proper balance for optimal health. For example, an excess of estrogen may lead to conditions like endometriosis, while low progesterone levels can affect fertility. Understanding these hormones and their functions helps women monitor their health and seek appropriate interventions when needed.

How Hormonal Imbalances Manifest (Symptoms and Signs)

Hormonal imbalances can present with various symptoms, such as irregular periods, weight gain or loss, mood swings, fatigue, and skin issues like acne or dryness. Women may also experience changes in libido and sleep disturbances. Recognizing these signs is crucial for identifying potential hormonal issues early.

Monitoring symptoms is the first step toward understanding and addressing hormonal imbalances. Keeping a journal of symptoms can help women identify patterns related to their cycles, stress levels, and lifestyle choices, allowing for better communication with healthcare providers about their hormonal health.

Factors Affecting Hormonal Balance (Diet, Stress, Environment)

Diet plays a significant role in hormonal balance, with certain foods promoting or hindering hormone production. For example, a diet rich in whole foods, healthy fats, and lean proteins supports optimal hormone function, while processed foods and sugars can lead to imbalances. Additionally, managing stress through mindfulness practices and regular exercise can help mitigate the adverse effects of stress hormones like cortisol.

Environmental factors, such as exposure to endocrine disruptors found in plastics and pesticides, can also impact hormonal health. Being mindful of the products used in daily life, opting for natural alternatives, and reducing exposure to harmful chemicals are practical steps to enhance hormonal balance.

The Menstrual Cycle and Its Hormonal Phases

The menstrual cycle consists of four phases: menstrual, follicular, ovulatory, and luteal. Each phase is characterized by specific hormonal changes. During the menstrual phase, estrogen and progesterone levels drop, leading to menstruation. The follicular phase sees rising estrogen levels, promoting egg maturation, while ovulation triggers a surge in estrogen and a spike in luteinizing hormone (LH).

Understanding these phases can help women track their cycles more effectively. By recognizing how hormone levels fluctuate throughout the cycle, women can better anticipate changes in mood, energy levels, and physical symptoms, facilitating more informed health decisions.

The Role of the Endocrine System in Hormone Regulation

The endocrine system comprises glands such as the pituitary, thyroid, and adrenal glands, which produce and regulate hormones throughout the body. This system works in concert to maintain hormonal balance and respond to various internal and external stimuli. For example, the hypothalamus in the brain regulates the pituitary gland, which in turn controls other glands and their hormone secretion.

To support a healthy endocrine system, women can prioritize a balanced diet, regular exercise, and adequate sleep. Incorporating practices such as yoga or meditation can also help manage stress, which is beneficial for maintaining hormonal health and overall well-being.

Common Misconceptions about Hormones

Many misconceptions about hormones persist, such as the belief that all hormonal changes are inherently negative or that only women experience hormonal imbalances. In reality, hormonal fluctuations are a natural part of life, influenced by various factors including age, lifestyle, and health conditions. Understanding that hormonal changes can be normal and expected is essential for women.

Education about hormones can empower women to seek appropriate care when necessary. By dispelling myths, individuals can foster a more informed approach to hormonal health, promoting better communication with healthcare providers and encouraging proactive management of their well-being.

The Impact of Aging on Hormone Levels

As women age, particularly during perimenopause and menopause, hormonal levels naturally decline, leading to various physical and emotional changes. This decline in estrogen and progesterone can result in symptoms such as hot flashes, mood swings, and changes in libido. It's essential to recognize these changes as a normal part of aging rather than a cause for concern.

To manage age-related hormonal changes, women can adopt lifestyle strategies such as regular exercise, a nutritious diet, and stress reduction techniques. These practices can help alleviate symptoms and improve overall health, making the transition through these life stages smoother and more manageable.

Understanding Hormone Testing and What to Look For

Hormone testing is crucial for identifying imbalances and understanding individual hormonal health.

Common tests include blood tests that measure levels of estrogen, progesterone, testosterone, and thyroid hormones. Women should consult healthcare professionals to determine which tests are appropriate based on their symptoms and health history.

Preparing for hormone testing involves being mindful of factors that may affect results, such as timing (certain tests may need to be taken at specific points in the menstrual cycle) and medication use. By being informed and proactive about testing, women can gain valuable insights into their hormonal health and take steps toward achieving balance.

Lifestyle Factors That Can Disrupt Hormonal Balance

Various lifestyle factors, such as poor diet, lack of exercise, and inadequate sleep, can disrupt hormonal balance. A diet high in refined sugars and unhealthy fats can lead to insulin resistance and inflammation, negatively impacting hormonal health. Regular physical activity, on the other hand, helps regulate hormones by improving insulin sensitivity and reducing stress levels.

Incorporating healthy habits such as meal prepping, engaging in regular physical activity, and prioritizing quality sleep can greatly improve hormonal balance. Simple changes, like swapping processed snacks for whole foods and establishing a bedtime routine, can lead to significant improvements in overall health and well-being.

Importance of Tracking Menstrual Cycles for Hormonal Health

Tracking menstrual cycles is vital for understanding hormonal health. By monitoring cycle length, flow, and associated symptoms, women can identify patterns and detect potential imbalances. This practice can also facilitate communication with healthcare providers, leading to more informed discussions about hormonal health and management strategies.

Women can utilize apps or journals to log their cycles and symptoms. Regular tracking helps women become more attuned to their bodies, allowing them to make proactive choices regarding their health and recognize when to seek medical advice.

Connection Between Hormonal Balance and Overall Well-Being

Hormonal balance is intricately connected to overall well-being. When hormones are in harmony, women often experience improved mood, energy levels, and reproductive health. Conversely, hormonal imbalances can lead to mental health issues, fatigue, and other health concerns, underscoring the importance of maintaining hormonal equilibrium.

To support overall well-being, women should adopt holistic approaches that encompass diet, exercise, stress management, and regular check-ups. By prioritizing these areas, women can foster hormonal health, enhancing their quality of life and emotional resilience.

Summary of Hormone Types Relevant to Women's Health

Key hormones relevant to women's health include estrogen, progesterone, testosterone, and cortisol. Each hormone serves distinct functions, such as regulating the menstrual cycle, influencing mood, and managing stress. Understanding these hormones helps women identify potential imbalances and recognize their impacts on overall health.

Being aware of hormone types and their functions empowers women to take charge of their health. By seeking appropriate testing, lifestyle modifications, and educational resources, women can effectively manage their hormonal health and enhance their well-being.

CHAPTER 2:

Nutrition for Hormonal Balance

Importance of a Balanced Diet for Hormonal Health

A balanced diet is crucial for maintaining hormonal health, as it provides the essential nutrients that the body needs to function optimally. Hormones are responsible for regulating many bodily processes, including metabolism, mood, and reproduction. When the body lacks essential nutrients, it can lead to hormonal imbalances, which may result in symptoms like fatigue, mood swings, and irregular menstrual cycles. Prioritizing a varied diet rich in whole foods ensures that your body receives the nutrients necessary for hormone production and regulation.

To achieve hormonal balance, focus on incorporating a variety of food groups into your daily meals. Aim for a plate that includes lean proteins, healthy fats, whole grains, and plenty of fruits and vegetables. This approach not only supports overall health but also provides the building blocks needed for hormone synthesis, helping to keep your hormonal levels stable and functioning efficiently.

Foods That Support Hormone Production

Certain foods are particularly beneficial for hormone production, helping to balance estrogen, progesterone, and testosterone levels. Healthy fats, such as those found in avocados, olive oil, and nuts, are vital for hormone synthesis and maintaining cell membranes. Protein sources like fish, eggs, and legumes provide amino acids essential for hormone formation. By incorporating these foods into your diet, you can enhance your body's ability to produce hormones effectively.

Additionally, don't overlook the importance of incorporating a range of micronutrients from whole foods. Foods rich in zinc (like pumpkin seeds), magnesium (found in leafy greens), and vitamins A, D, and E (from eggs and dairy) are crucial for hormone production. By prioritizing these foods, you can support your body's hormonal balance naturally.

Nutrient Deficiencies That Can Affect Hormone Levels

Nutrient deficiencies can significantly impact hormone levels and overall health. For example, deficiencies in vitamins D and B6, magnesium, and zinc are linked to hormonal imbalances that can lead to irregular menstrual cycles and mood disorders. Identifying and addressing these deficiencies through diet or supplementation is crucial for restoring balance and preventing complications.

To avoid these deficiencies, regularly include foods rich in these essential nutrients in your diet. For instance, incorporate leafy greens, nuts, seeds, fatty fish, and fortified foods to ensure you meet your daily requirements. If you suspect a deficiency, consider consulting a healthcare provider to get tailored advice and potential supplementation.

Role of Fiber in Hormone Regulation

Fiber plays a vital role in regulating hormones by promoting gut health and aiding in the elimination of excess hormones from the body. A high-fiber diet supports healthy digestion and can help to prevent hormonal fluctuations that may lead to weight gain or mood swings. Soluble fiber, found in foods like oats, beans, and fruits, can help stabilize blood sugar levels, which is crucial for hormone regulation.

To increase your fiber intake, aim for at least 25-30 grams per day by incorporating whole grains, fruits, vegetables, and legumes into your meals. Starting your day with oatmeal, snacking on fruits, and including a variety of vegetables at lunch and dinner are practical ways to boost fiber in your diet while supporting hormonal health.

Hydration's Impact on Hormonal Health

Staying adequately hydrated is essential for maintaining hormonal balance, as water plays a crucial role in many bodily functions, including hormone transport and metabolic processes. Dehydration can lead to symptoms such as fatigue, irritability, and concentration difficulties, which can be exacerbated by hormonal imbalances. Aim to drink at least 8-10 cups of water daily, adjusting based on activity level and climate.

To enhance your hydration, consider incorporating water-rich foods like fruits and vegetables into your diet, such as cucumbers, oranges, and watermelon. Additionally, herbal teas can be a soothing way to increase fluid intake. Monitoring your hydration status can be as simple as checking the color of your urine—aim for a light yellow shade as an indicator of good hydration.

Anti-Inflammatory Foods to Include in Your Diet

Incorporating anti-inflammatory foods into your diet can significantly benefit hormonal health by reducing chronic inflammation, which is linked to hormonal imbalances. Foods rich in omega-3 fatty acids, such as fatty fish (salmon, mackerel), flaxseeds, and walnuts, are excellent choices. Additionally, colorful fruits and vegetables, like berries and leafy greens, provide antioxidants that help combat inflammation.

To integrate these foods into your meals, consider preparing a salmon salad with mixed greens and berries for lunch, or snack on walnuts and carrot sticks for a nutritious boost. Regularly including these anti-inflammatory foods can help promote hormonal balance and overall well-being.

Foods to Avoid for Better Hormonal Balance

Certain foods can disrupt hormonal balance and contribute to imbalances. High sugar intake and heavily processed foods can lead to insulin resistance and inflammation, negatively affecting hormone levels. Additionally, trans fats found in fried and packaged foods may contribute to hormonal dysregulation. Minimizing these foods in your diet is essential for maintaining hormonal health.

To promote better hormonal balance, focus on reducing sugar-laden snacks and opting for whole, unprocessed foods. Instead of reaching for a candy bar, try a piece of fruit or a handful of nuts for a satisfying snack. Being mindful of your food choices can help you support your hormonal health effectively.

How to Incorporate Phytoestrogens Into Your Diet

Phytoestrogens are plant compounds that mimic estrogen in the body and can help balance hormone levels. Foods rich in phytoestrogens include soy products (tofu, tempeh), flaxseeds, sesame seeds, and whole grains. Including these foods in your diet can provide a natural way to support hormonal balance, especially during menopause or hormonal fluctuations.

To incorporate phytoestrogens into your meals, try adding flaxseeds to smoothies, using tofu in stir-fries, or enjoying a sesame seed topping on salads. These small dietary changes can make a significant difference in supporting hormone levels and overall wellness.

The Benefits of a Mediterranean Diet for Women

The Mediterranean diet emphasizes whole foods, healthy fats, and plenty of fruits and vegetables, making it particularly beneficial for women's hormonal health. Rich in omega-3 fatty acids, antioxidants, and fiber, this diet supports overall health while helping to regulate hormones. Studies have shown that adherence to a Mediterranean diet can lead to improved metabolic health and reduced symptoms of hormonal imbalance.

To start following a Mediterranean diet, focus on incorporating more olive oil, fish, whole grains, and fresh produce into your meals. Planning meals that highlight these components—like a grilled fish with quinoa and roasted vegetables—can create delicious and healthful dishes that support hormonal balance.

Meal Planning Tips for Balanced Nutrition

Meal planning is an effective strategy to ensure you maintain balanced nutrition for hormonal health. Start by setting aside time each week to plan your meals, making a grocery list that includes a variety of whole foods, proteins, healthy fats, and plenty of fruits and vegetables. This preparation will help you make healthier choices and avoid last-minute unhealthy options.

When planning meals, consider batch cooking and preparing snacks in advance to save time during the week. For example, cook a large batch of quinoa and roast a variety of vegetables to have on hand for easy meal assembly. This approach not only saves time but also helps you stay committed to a balanced diet.

The Significance of Timing Your Meals

Timing your meals can have a significant impact on hormonal balance. For many women, intermittent fasting—a pattern of eating where you cycle between periods of eating and fasting—can help improve insulin sensitivity and regulate hormonal fluctuations. Aim for a schedule that works for you, such as eating within an 8-hour window and fasting for the remaining 16 hours.

To implement meal timing effectively, begin by gradually adjusting your eating schedule. For instance, if you usually eat breakfast at 8 AM, try delaying it to 10 AM. This adjustment can help your body adapt to a new rhythm, potentially improving hormonal balance and overall energy levels.

The Impact of Caffeine and Alcohol on Hormones

Caffeine and alcohol can significantly affect hormonal health when consumed in excess. High caffeine intake can lead to increased cortisol levels, potentially causing stress and disrupting hormonal balance. Similarly, alcohol can interfere with hormone metabolism, leading to imbalances and negative health effects. Moderation is key; aim to limit caffeine to one or two servings per day and consider reducing alcohol consumption.

To minimize the impact of these substances, replace your regular coffee with herbal teas or opt for decaffeinated versions when possible. If you choose to drink alcohol, consider setting limits, such as only enjoying it on weekends or special occasions, which can help maintain hormonal stability and improve overall wellness.

The Importance of Micronutrients for Hormonal Health

Micronutrients, including vitamins and minerals, are essential for hormonal health as they play crucial roles in hormone production and regulation. Vitamins like B6, D, and E, along with minerals such as magnesium and zinc, are particularly important for maintaining hormonal balance. A deficiency in these micronutrients can lead to issues like mood swings, fatigue, and irregular cycles.

To ensure you are getting enough micronutrients, focus on consuming a varied diet rich in fruits, vegetables, whole grains, nuts, and seeds. If you find it challenging to meet your micronutrient needs through food alone, consider discussing supplementation options with a healthcare professional to support your hormonal health effectively.

CHAPTER 3:

Stress Management Techniques

Understanding the Connection between Stress and Hormones

Stress triggers the release of hormones like cortisol and adrenaline, which prepare the body for a fight-or-flight response. Chronic stress can lead to hormonal imbalances that disrupt menstrual cycles, increase fatigue, and heighten anxiety. To understand this connection, pay attention to how you feel during stressful situations and note any changes in your body or mood. Recognizing these patterns is the first step in managing stress and restoring hormonal balance.

To counteract stress's effects on hormones, aim to incorporate stress-reducing practices into your daily life. Begin by monitoring your stress levels and their impact on your health. Awareness allows you to identify when you are feeling overwhelmed, helping you to respond proactively before stress escalates into chronic issues.

Identifying Sources of Stress in Daily Life

Begin by keeping a stress diary for at least a week. Document situations that trigger stress, your reactions, and any physical sensations you experience. This practice helps pinpoint patterns, whether they stem from work, relationships, or financial concerns, and allows you to see where you might need to make changes.

Once you've identified your stress sources, consider practical steps to address them. For example, if work deadlines are a major stressor, break tasks into smaller, manageable chunks. Communicate with colleagues or seek support to create a more manageable workload, reducing the overall pressure you feel.

Effective Stress Reduction Techniques

Practicing meditation can significantly reduce stress by promoting relaxation and enhancing emotional clarity.

Start with just five minutes a day, focusing on your breath or a simple mantra. Gradually increase the time as you become more comfortable. Consider using guided meditations through apps or online resources to help establish a routine.

Deep breathing exercises are another effective technique. Take a moment to close your eyes and breathe in deeply through your nose, allowing your abdomen to expand. Hold for a few seconds, then exhale slowly through your mouth. Repeat this for several cycles, focusing on the calming sensation of your breath to ease stress and ground yourself in the present moment.

The Role of Exercise in Managing Stress Levels

Physical activity is a powerful way to combat stress and regulate hormones. Aim for at least 30 minutes of moderate exercise most days of the week, whether it's brisk walking, dancing, or yoga. Exercise releases endorphins, which boost mood and alleviate feelings of stress.

Incorporate activities you enjoy into your routine to stay motivated. Schedule workouts into your calendar as you would any important appointment, ensuring you dedicate time to your physical and mental well-being. Even short bursts of movement throughout the day can help maintain lower stress levels and improve your overall mood.

Importance of Sleep for Hormonal Balance

Quality sleep is crucial for maintaining hormonal balance. Aim for 7-9 hours of sleep per night by establishing a consistent sleep schedule. Go to bed and wake up at the same time each day, even on weekends, to regulate your body's internal clock.

Create a restful environment by minimizing distractions. Dim the lights in the evening, keep electronics out of the bedroom, and consider incorporating a relaxing pre-sleep routine such as reading or taking a warm bath. Prioritizing sleep helps your body restore hormonal balance, reduces stress, and enhances overall wellness.

Techniques for Creating a Relaxing Environment

Transform your space into a sanctuary by decluttering and organizing. A clean and orderly environment can significantly reduce stress. Incorporate soothing elements like soft lighting, calming colors, and comfortable furniture to create a welcoming atmosphere.

Adding natural elements such as plants or aromatherapy can also enhance relaxation. Consider using essential oils like lavender or chamomile in a diffuser to promote calmness. Make your space a haven where you can unwind and recharge, allowing for greater resilience against daily stressors.

The Benefits of Mindfulness Practices

Mindfulness practices, such as yoga and meditation, encourage awareness of the present moment, helping to reduce anxiety and improve emotional regulation. Start by dedicating a few minutes each day to simply observe your thoughts and feelings without judgment. This practice cultivates a greater understanding of your emotional responses and reduces stress.

Incorporate mindfulness into daily activities, such as eating or walking. Focus on the sensations, flavors, or sounds you experience, which fosters a sense of calm and presence. Over time, these practices can enhance your ability to handle stressors more effectively.

Setting Healthy Boundaries to Reduce Stress

Establishing healthy boundaries is vital for protecting your time and energy. Begin by identifying areas in your life where you feel overwhelmed or taken advantage of.

Communicate your needs clearly and assertively to those around you, whether at work or in personal relationships.

Practice saying no when necessary, ensuring you do not overcommit yourself. Remember that setting boundaries is not selfish; it is a crucial step toward maintaining your well-being and preventing burnout. Healthy boundaries empower you to prioritize your mental health.

The Role of Social Support in Stress Management

Having a strong social support network can significantly reduce stress. Identify friends, family, or support groups that you can turn to when you're feeling overwhelmed. Regularly connect with these individuals, whether through phone calls, text messages, or in-person meet-ups, to foster these supportive relationships.

Engage in open conversations about your feelings and challenges. Sharing your experiences not only provides emotional relief but also strengthens bonds with others.

Building and maintaining a supportive network is essential for managing stress and enhancing overall wellness

Utilizing Journaling for Emotional Release

Journaling can serve as a powerful tool for processing emotions and relieving stress. Set aside time each day or week to write about your thoughts, feelings, and experiences. Don't worry about grammar or structure; focus instead on expressing your emotions honestly.

Consider incorporating prompts to guide your writing. Questions like "What am I grateful for today?" or "What challenges did I face?" can help you reflect and gain perspective. Regular journaling not only promotes emotional release but also helps you identify patterns in your thoughts and behaviors.

The Importance of Hobbies and Leisure Activities

Engaging in hobbies and leisure activities is essential for maintaining a balanced and fulfilling life. Dedicate time each week to activities you enjoy, whether it's painting, gardening, or playing a musical instrument. These activities serve as an outlet for creativity and relaxation.

Make it a priority to disconnect from responsibilities during this time. Allow yourself to fully immerse in your chosen activity without distractions. This practice can significantly reduce stress and enhance your overall sense of well-being.

How to Recognize Burnout and Take Preventive Measures

Recognizing the signs of burnout is crucial for maintaining mental health. Symptoms can include chronic fatigue, irritability, and decreased productivity. Pay attention to your physical and emotional state, noting when you feel overwhelmed or disengaged from your usual activities.

To prevent burnout, establish a self-care routine that includes regular breaks, healthy boundaries, and activities that bring you joy. Schedule time for relaxation and ensure you're not overcommitting to work or other obligations. Prioritizing your well-being helps protect against burnout and promotes overall health.

Building a Stress Management Routine That Works for You

Creating a personalized stress management routine involves identifying the techniques that resonate most with you. Start by experimenting with various practices, such as meditation, exercise, or journaling, to discover what brings you the most relief. Reflect on your experiences and adjust your routine based on what feels effective.

Incorporate these practices into your daily or weekly schedule, treating them as essential appointments for your well-being. Consistency is key to seeing lasting benefits, so commit to prioritizing your stress management routine and remain open to making changes as needed for optimal results.

CHAPTER 4:

Exercise and Hormonal Health

Benefits of Physical Activity for Hormone Balance

Engaging in regular physical activity is essential for maintaining hormonal balance. Exercise stimulates the release of various hormones, such as insulin, cortisol, and endorphins, which play vital roles in mood regulation, stress management, and metabolic processes. By incorporating physical activity into your routine, you can help mitigate symptoms related to hormonal imbalances, such as mood swings, fatigue, and weight gain.

To maximize these benefits, aim for at least 150 minutes of moderate aerobic activity or 75 minutes of vigorous activity each week. This could include brisk walking, cycling, swimming, or any enjoyable activity that gets your heart rate up. Additionally, incorporating strength training at least twice a week can further enhance hormonal health by building muscle mass, which improves metabolism and insulin sensitivity.

Different Types of Exercise and Their Effects on Hormones

Different forms of exercise can uniquely influence hormone levels in the body. Strength training, for example, is known to increase testosterone and growth hormone, promoting muscle growth and fat loss. In contrast, cardiovascular exercise primarily impacts insulin sensitivity and helps regulate cortisol levels, providing a stress-relieving effect that can balance hormones.

To create a comprehensive exercise regimen, combine both strength training and cardio. For instance, you might alternate between weightlifting sessions and cardio workouts like jogging or cycling throughout the week. This approach ensures that you benefit from the various hormonal responses triggered by each type of exercise.

The Importance of Regular Movement in Daily Life

Incorporating regular movement into your daily routine is crucial for maintaining hormone balance. Simple activities such as walking, stretching, or even gardening can significantly impact your overall well-being. These small changes can enhance blood circulation, promote the release of feel-good hormones, and improve energy levels.

To make movement a part of your daily life, consider setting reminders to take short breaks for stretching or walking. Additionally, choose active transportation methods, such as walking or cycling instead of driving, to naturally integrate movement into your day-to-day activities.

How to Create a Balanced Exercise Routine

A balanced exercise routine combines various forms of physical activity to promote overall hormonal health.

Start by assessing your fitness level and identifying your goals, such as weight loss, strength building, or improved endurance. Then, create a schedule that includes a mix of cardio, strength training, and flexibility exercises, ensuring you address all aspects of fitness.

Aim to work out at least three to five times per week, dedicating specific days to each type of exercise. For example, you could designate Monday and Thursday for strength training, Tuesday and Friday for cardio, and Wednesday for flexibility and mobility work. This variety will keep your routine engaging and provide comprehensive benefits for hormone balance.

Recognizing When to Rest and Recover

Rest and recovery are crucial components of a successful exercise routine, especially for hormonal balance. Overtraining can lead to increased cortisol levels, fatigue, and mood disturbances, which can negatively impact your hormones. It's essential to listen to your body and recognize signs of overexertion, such as persistent soreness, irritability, or sleep disturbances.

To ensure adequate recovery, incorporate rest days into your exercise routine and prioritize sleep. This could mean taking one or two days off from intense workouts or engaging in lighter activities like walking or yoga on recovery days. By giving your body time to heal, you can maintain optimal hormonal function and prevent burnout.

The Impact of Overtraining on Hormonal Health

Overtraining can severely affect hormonal health, leading to elevated cortisol levels and hormonal imbalances. This stress response can manifest as fatigue, disrupted sleep patterns, and mood fluctuations. To mitigate these effects, it's crucial to balance exercise intensity with adequate rest and recovery.

If you suspect you're experiencing symptoms of overtraining, consider reevaluating your exercise routine. Implementing lighter workouts, increasing rest days, and focusing on recovery strategies such as proper nutrition and hydration can help restore hormonal balance and improve your overall health.

Fun Ways to Incorporate Movement into Your Day

Incorporating movement into your daily routine doesn't have to feel like a chore. Find enjoyable activities that get you moving, such as dancing, hiking, or playing a sport. Engaging in fun activities can boost your mood and motivation while providing significant benefits for your hormonal health.

To make it even easier, consider scheduling these activities with friends or family. Social engagement can enhance your experience and encourage you to stay active consistently. Look for local classes or community events that align with your interests to keep the momentum going.

Exploring Yoga and Its Benefits for Hormonal Balance

Yoga is a powerful tool for promoting hormonal balance through mindful movement and breath work. Various poses can stimulate the endocrine system, aiding in the regulation of hormones such as estrogen and progesterone. Additionally, the practice emphasizes relaxation and stress relief, helping to lower cortisol levels and improve overall well-being.

To incorporate yoga into your routine, start with beginner classes or online tutorials. Aim for at least two to three sessions per week, focusing on poses that encourage relaxation and flexibility, such as Child's Pose or Downward Dog. With regular practice, you may notice improved mood, reduced stress, and enhanced hormonal balance.

Understanding the Role of Endorphins in Mood Regulation

Endorphins are hormones released during physical activity that contribute to feelings of happiness and well-being. Engaging in regular exercise can significantly increase endorphin levels, helping to alleviate symptoms of stress, anxiety, and depression. This natural mood boost is essential for maintaining a balanced hormonal profile.

To harness the power of endorphins, choose activities that you enjoy and that challenge you. Whether it's running, dancing, or engaging in a sport, find what works for you. Aim to incorporate at least 30 minutes of moderate-intensity exercise most days of the week to maximize endorphin release and support your emotional health.

Finding Activities That You Enjoy to Stay Motivated

Staying active becomes much easier when you engage in activities that you genuinely enjoy. Experiment with different forms of exercise to discover what resonates with you, whether it's group classes, outdoor activities, or individual sports. Finding joy in movement can help you maintain consistency and reap the benefits for hormonal balance.

To stay motivated, consider setting personal challenges or joining a community group related to your chosen activity. This support can keep you engaged and encourage you to stick with your fitness journey, ultimately leading to better hormone regulation and overall health.

Tips for Setting Achievable Fitness Goals

Setting achievable fitness goals is essential for maintaining motivation and tracking progress. Start by defining your objectives, such as improving endurance, building strength, or losing weight. Use the SMART criteria—Specific, Measurable, Achievable, Relevant, and Time-bound—to create clear and realistic goals.

Break your larger goals into smaller, manageable steps. For example, if your aim is to run a 5K, start by setting milestones like running for 10 minutes without stopping or gradually increasing your distance each week. Celebrating these small victories can boost your confidence and commitment to your fitness journey.

Importance of Flexibility and Mobility Exercises

Flexibility and mobility exercises play a vital role in maintaining overall health and hormonal balance. Regular stretching can enhance blood flow, reduce muscle tension, and improve your range of motion, all of which contribute to better performance during physical activity. This can ultimately influence hormone regulation by reducing stress and supporting overall well-being.

Incorporate flexibility and mobility exercises into your routine at least two to three times a week. Consider activities such as yoga, Pilates, or dedicated stretching sessions. Focus on areas that may feel tight or restricted, and prioritize deep breathing to further enhance relaxation and stress relief.

The Relationship Between Body Composition and Hormone Levels

Body composition significantly influences hormone levels and overall hormonal health. Higher body fat percentages can lead to elevated estrogen levels, potentially resulting in hormonal imbalances. Conversely, maintaining a healthy body composition through balanced nutrition and regular exercise can help regulate hormones effectively.

To support healthy body composition, focus on whole, nutrient-dense foods while incorporating regular physical activity. Aim to combine cardiovascular exercise, strength training, and flexibility work in your routine.

CHAPTER 5:

Natural Remedies for Hormonal Balance

Overview of Herbal Supplements that Support Hormonal Health

Herbal supplements can play a significant role in supporting hormonal balance for women. Popular options include **vitex (chaste tree)**, which may help regulate the menstrual cycle, and **black cohosh**, often used to ease menopausal symptoms. Other effective herbs include **dong quai**, known for its blood-building properties, and **ashwagandha**, which can aid in managing stress levels. It's essential to explore these herbs through reputable sources to ensure the right selection for your specific hormonal needs.

To incorporate herbal supplements into your routine, start by assessing your hormonal symptoms and researching suitable options. Consulting with a healthcare provider who specializes in herbal medicine can guide you in choosing the right supplements. Begin with low doses to observe how your body responds, and consider keeping a journal to track your symptoms and any changes. This practice will help you make informed decisions about continuing or adjusting your supplement regimen.

The Role of Essential Oils in Balancing Hormones

Essential oils can be powerful allies in hormonal balance, offering therapeutic benefits through their natural properties. Oils like **lavender** and **clary sage** have calming effects that may help alleviate stress and hormonal fluctuations. Additionally, **geranium** oil is believed to help regulate estrogen levels, making it beneficial during the menstrual cycle or menopause. To use essential oils, you can diffuse them in your home, add them to a warm bath, or mix with a carrier oil for topical application.

When using essential oils, it's crucial to select high-quality, pure products to ensure effectiveness and safety. Start with a few drops in a diffuser or diluted in a carrier oil for massage. Be mindful of any skin sensitivities by conducting a patch test before full application. If you're pregnant or nursing, consult a healthcare professional before using essential oils, as some may not be suitable during these times.

Benefits of Acupuncture and Traditional Therapies

Acupuncture, a traditional Chinese medicine practice, has gained recognition for its potential benefits in balancing hormones and alleviating related symptoms. By inserting fine needles into specific points on the body, acupuncture is believed to stimulate energy flow, which can help regulate hormonal cycles and reduce menstrual pain. Many women have reported improvements in symptoms of PMS and menopause, making it a viable option for those seeking natural relief.

To explore acupuncture, seek out licensed practitioners who have experience with women's health issues. During your first appointment, you'll discuss your specific symptoms and health history. Treatments typically involve a series of sessions, often ranging from weekly to bi-weekly, depending on individual needs. Combining acupuncture with other holistic practices, such as herbal therapy or nutritional adjustments, can enhance overall effectiveness.

Exploring the Impact of Adaptogens on Stress Hormones

Adaptogens are natural substances that help the body adapt to stress and promote hormonal balance. Herbs like **rhodiola**, **holy basil**, and **ginseng** are known for their ability to support the adrenal glands, which regulate stress hormones like cortisol. By incorporating adaptogens into your daily routine, you may experience reduced anxiety, improved mood, and enhanced energy levels, making them an effective option for women facing hormonal imbalances due to stress.

To utilize adaptogens, start by selecting a few that resonate with you and researching their effects. These can be consumed as teas, capsules, or powders mixed into smoothies. It's essential to monitor your body's response and consult with a healthcare provider if you have any underlying health conditions or are taking medications, as some adaptogens may interact with other treatments.

Foods as Medicine: Using Spices for Hormonal Health

Integrating specific spices into your diet can significantly enhance hormonal health. Spices like **turmeric**, which contains curcumin, have anti-inflammatory properties that may support hormonal balance. **Cinnamon** can help regulate blood sugar levels, which is crucial for maintaining stable energy and hormonal function. Additionally, **fenugreek** seeds are known to have potential benefits in balancing estrogen levels and promoting reproductive health.

To incorporate these spices into your meals, start by adding turmeric and cinnamon to your morning smoothie or oatmeal. Fenugreek can be used in cooking or brewed as a tea. Aim to include a variety of these spices in your daily diet to experience their full benefits. Keeping a food diary can help track your intake and its effects on your hormonal health over time.

Importance of Consulting with Healthcare Professionals

Consulting with healthcare professionals is vital when exploring natural hormone balancing methods. A qualified practitioner can help assess your hormonal health through comprehensive testing and personalized recommendations. They can also provide guidance on appropriate supplements, essential oils, and lifestyle changes that align with your specific needs, ensuring that your approach is safe and effective.

When seeking a healthcare professional, look for those with experience in integrative or holistic medicine, as they are often more familiar with natural therapies. Preparing for your appointment by noting your symptoms, medical history, and questions can lead to a more productive discussion. Regular check-ins with your healthcare provider will help you monitor your progress and make necessary adjustments to your treatment plan.

How to Safely Use Supplements and Remedies

Using supplements and natural remedies safely requires careful consideration and proper guidance. Start by conducting thorough research on the supplements you're interested in, focusing on reputable brands and high-quality products. It's important to follow dosage recommendations and be aware of any potential interactions with medications you may be taking.

Before starting any new supplement, consider consulting with a healthcare professional, especially if you have pre-existing health conditions or are pregnant. Keeping a journal to track your symptoms and any side effects can help you gauge the effectiveness of the supplements. If you experience any adverse reactions, discontinue use immediately and consult your healthcare provider.

Understanding the Research behind Natural Treatments

Understanding the research surrounding natural treatments for hormonal balance is essential for making informed choices. Many studies highlight the efficacy of herbs, essential oils, and dietary changes in promoting hormonal health. It's crucial to look for peer-reviewed studies and reputable sources when researching these treatments to ensure they are backed by solid evidence.

To stay informed, consider subscribing to reputable health journals, attending workshops, or participating in online courses focusing on women's health and natural remedies. Engaging in discussions with healthcare providers knowledgeable about the latest research can also enhance your understanding and help you apply evidence-based practices to your wellness journey.

The Significance of Holistic Practitioners in Care

Holistic practitioners play a vital role in women's health by addressing the interconnectedness of body, mind, and spirit. They often utilize a combination of conventional medicine and alternative therapies to create personalized treatment plans. By taking into account lifestyle factors, emotional well-being, and nutritional habits, holistic practitioners can provide comprehensive care tailored to your individual needs.

To benefit from holistic care, seek practitioners who are certified and have experience in integrative approaches. During your initial consultation, discuss your health concerns and goals, and inquire about the various therapies they offer. Building a trusting relationship with your holistic practitioner can lead to better health outcomes and a more fulfilling wellness journey.

Assessing the Quality of Herbal Products

Assessing the quality of herbal products is essential to ensure safety and effectiveness. Look for supplements that are third-party tested for purity and potency, as these certifications indicate that the product has been independently evaluated. Additionally, opt for brands that provide transparency about their sourcing and manufacturing processes.

To further ensure quality, check for standardized extracts, which guarantee consistent levels of active ingredients. Read customer reviews and research any reported side effects to gauge the product's reliability. By prioritizing high-quality herbal products, you can enhance your chances of achieving hormonal balance through natural means.

The Potential Risks and Side Effects of Natural Remedies

While natural remedies can be beneficial, they also carry potential risks and side effects that should not be overlooked. Some herbal supplements can interact with prescription medications, potentially diminishing their effectiveness or causing adverse reactions. For instance, **St. John's Wort** can interfere with antidepressants, and **ginkgo biloba** may affect blood clotting.

To mitigate these risks, always inform your healthcare provider about any natural remedies you're considering. Start with lower doses to observe how your body reacts, and keep a record of any side effects you experience. If you encounter unexpected reactions, discontinue use and consult your healthcare provider for guidance on alternative options.

Creating a Personalized Natural Health Plan

Creating a personalized natural health plan involves assessing your unique health needs and lifestyle factors. Start by identifying your hormonal symptoms and lifestyle habits that may contribute to imbalances. This can include stress levels, diet, exercise, and sleep patterns.

Once you have a clear picture of your health landscape, set specific, achievable goals for hormonal balance. Incorporate a mix of dietary adjustments, supplements, and stress-management techniques into your plan. Regularly review and adjust your health plan based on your progress and any changes in symptoms to ensure it continues to meet your needs effectively.

Combining Natural Remedies with Conventional Medicine

Combining natural remedies with conventional medicine can enhance overall wellness while promoting hormonal balance. It's important to approach this integration thoughtfully, ensuring that both practices complement each other rather than conflict. Open communication with your healthcare provider about your use of natural remedies is essential to create a cohesive treatment strategy.

To start combining approaches, begin with one or two natural remedies and monitor your body's response alongside any conventional treatments. Discuss potential interactions and side effects with your healthcare provider to tailor your approach. This collaborative method allows for a more holistic treatment plan that supports your health goals while minimizing risks.

CHAPTER 6:

Hormonal Imbalances and Their Impact

Common Hormonal Imbalances in Women (e.g., PCOS, Menopause)

Hormonal imbalances in women can manifest in various forms, with conditions like Polycystic Ovary Syndrome (PCOS) and menopause being among the most common. PCOS is characterized by irregular menstrual cycles, excessive hair growth, and weight gain due to elevated androgen levels, while menopause marks the end of menstruation, often leading to symptoms like hot flashes and mood changes. Identifying these conditions early can significantly improve management and overall well-being.

To manage these imbalances, it's essential to consult a healthcare provider for proper diagnosis and treatment options. Lifestyle changes, including diet and exercise, can be beneficial, as well as tracking your menstrual cycle and any symptoms you experience to share with your doctor. Understanding your body and its hormonal rhythms is the first step towards achieving balance.

Understanding Symptoms and Their Implications

Recognizing the symptoms of hormonal imbalance is crucial for taking proactive steps towards wellness. Common symptoms include irregular periods, fatigue, mood swings, weight changes, and skin issues. Each of these indicators can have broader implications, such as affecting your fertility, energy levels, and mental health.

Keeping a symptom diary can help you identify patterns and triggers. Note when symptoms occur, their severity, and any related lifestyle factors. This information can assist healthcare providers in developing a tailored treatment plan to address your specific needs.

The Connection Between Hormonal Imbalance and Mental Health

Hormonal imbalances can significantly impact mental health, often leading to mood disorders such as anxiety and depression. Fluctuating estrogen and progesterone levels can influence neurotransmitters in the brain, affecting your emotional well-being. Understanding this connection is vital for women experiencing mood swings or mental health challenges.

To address these issues, consider incorporating stress-reduction techniques into your daily routine, such as mindfulness, yoga, or meditation. Additionally, maintaining a balanced diet rich in omega-3 fatty acids, whole grains, and leafy greens can support brain health and stabilize mood.

How Hormonal Issues Can Affect Weight and Metabolism

Hormonal imbalances can disrupt metabolic processes, leading to weight gain or difficulty losing weight. For instance, insulin resistance often associated with PCOS can hinder the body's ability to process sugars efficiently, contributing to weight gain. Additionally, thyroid issues can lower metabolism, making it challenging to maintain a healthy weight.

To combat these effects, focus on a balanced diet that prioritizes whole foods and healthy fats while minimizing processed foods and sugars. Regular exercise is equally important; incorporate both cardiovascular activities and strength training to boost metabolism and support weight management.

Exploring Fertility Challenges Related to Hormone Levels

Hormonal imbalances can pose significant challenges to fertility, affecting ovulation and menstrual regularity. Conditions like PCOS and thyroid disorders can interfere with hormone production, making conception more difficult. Understanding how these hormones work can empower women to seek appropriate interventions.

For women facing fertility issues, tracking ovulation through methods such as basal body temperature monitoring or ovulation predictor kits can be helpful. Consulting a fertility specialist can provide targeted treatments, including hormonal therapies or lifestyle changes to optimize chances of conception.

The Role of Hormones in Skin Health and Aging

Hormones play a crucial role in maintaining skin health, influencing moisture, elasticity, and overall appearance. Estrogen, for example, helps maintain skin thickness and hydration, while a drop in hormone levels during menopause can lead to dryness and wrinkles. Understanding these changes can guide appropriate skincare choices.

To support skin health, adopt a skincare routine that includes moisturizing products and antioxidants. Additionally, consider dietary choices rich in vitamins A, C, and E, which promote skin regeneration. Staying hydrated and protecting your skin from sun damage can also combat aging effects.

The Impact of Hormonal Imbalances on Sleep Patterns

Hormonal imbalances can disrupt sleep patterns, often leading to insomnia or poor sleep quality. Fluctuations in hormones like progesterone and cortisol can affect sleep cycles, causing night sweats or difficulty falling asleep. Recognizing the impact of hormones on sleep is essential for addressing these challenges.

To improve sleep quality, establish a regular bedtime routine, limiting screen time before bed and creating a calming environment. Incorporating relaxation techniques such as deep breathing or light yoga can also help promote better sleep, along with avoiding caffeine and heavy meals close to bedtime.

Connection Between Hormonal Health and Chronic Conditions

Hormonal health is intricately linked to various chronic conditions, including diabetes, heart disease, and autoimmune disorders. Imbalances can exacerbate these conditions or lead to new health challenges. Understanding this relationship can encourage proactive management and prevention strategies.

Regular check-ups and screenings are vital for monitoring hormonal health, particularly if you have a family history of chronic conditions. Maintaining a balanced diet, exercising regularly, and managing stress can also contribute to reducing the risk of developing these health issues.

When to Seek Medical Advice for Hormonal Issues

Recognizing when to seek medical advice is essential for effective management of hormonal imbalances. If you experience persistent symptoms such as extreme fatigue, irregular periods, or severe mood swings, it's important to consult a healthcare provider. Early intervention can lead to more effective treatment options.

During your visit, be prepared to discuss your symptoms, medical history, and any lifestyle factors that may contribute to hormonal issues. A thorough evaluation, including blood tests and possibly imaging, can help pinpoint the underlying causes and lead to a tailored treatment plan.

Overview of Conventional Treatments Available

Conventional treatments for hormonal imbalances often include hormone replacement therapy (HRT), medications to regulate menstrual cycles, and insulin-sensitizing agents for conditions like PCOS. These treatments aim to restore hormonal balance and alleviate symptoms. Understanding available options empowers women to make informed decisions about their health.

Consulting with a healthcare provider specializing in hormonal health can provide guidance on the most suitable treatment for your specific situation. Regular follow-ups are crucial to monitor effectiveness and adjust treatments as necessary for optimal results.

The Importance of Regular Check-Ups for Hormonal Health

Regular check-ups play a vital role in maintaining hormonal health, allowing for early detection of imbalances or related conditions. These visits provide opportunities to discuss symptoms, receive screenings, and adjust any ongoing treatments. Proactive healthcare can lead to improved well-being and reduced risk of complications.

To prioritize your hormonal health, schedule annual check-ups and stay consistent with any recommended screenings. Preparing for your appointments by tracking symptoms and asking questions can help you make the most of your time with your healthcare provider.

Recognizing the Need for Lifestyle Changes

Lifestyle changes are often essential for restoring hormonal balance and enhancing overall wellness. Factors such as diet, exercise, stress management, and sleep can significantly impact hormonal health. Recognizing areas for improvement can empower women to take actionable steps toward better health.

Start by incorporating nutrient-dense foods into your diet, engaging in regular physical activity, and practicing stress-reducing techniques. Small changes, such as taking walks, cooking at home, or practicing mindfulness, can create lasting improvements in your hormonal health.

Encouragement for Women to Advocate for Their Health

Women are encouraged to advocate for their health, especially concerning hormonal issues. Taking an active role in your healthcare by educating yourself about hormonal health, asking questions, and expressing concerns can lead to better outcomes. Empowerment through knowledge is crucial for effective management.

Joining support groups or seeking information from credible sources can provide additional insights and encouragement. By sharing experiences and strategies with others, women can foster a community of support that prioritizes hormonal health and overall well-being.

CHAPTER 7:

The Role of Sleep in Hormonal Balance

Understanding How Sleep Affects Hormone Production

Sleep plays a crucial role in hormone production, particularly in regulating hormones such as cortisol, melatonin, and growth hormone. During deep sleep stages, the body undergoes vital restorative processes that help in hormone synthesis. For women, this is particularly important as fluctuations in hormone levels can significantly impact menstrual cycles, fertility, and overall health.

To optimize hormone production, aim for 7-9 hours of quality sleep each night. Establishing a consistent sleep schedule helps regulate your body's internal clock, ensuring that hormone levels remain stable. Tracking your sleep patterns using apps or journals can also provide insights into your sleep quality and help identify areas for improvement.

The Importance of Quality Sleep for Women's Health

Quality sleep is fundamental for maintaining women's health as it supports physical, mental, and emotional well-being. During sleep, the body repairs tissues, regulates metabolism, and balances hormones, making it essential for functions like immune response and mood stability. Poor sleep quality can lead to imbalances in hormones such as estrogen and progesterone, affecting menstrual health and increasing the risk of conditions like polycystic ovary syndrome (PCOS).

To prioritize quality sleep, focus on creating a soothing bedtime atmosphere. This can include dimming lights, avoiding stimulating activities before bed, and establishing a comfortable temperature in your bedroom. Consider investing in high-quality bedding to further enhance your sleep environment.

Common Sleep Disorders That Impact Hormones

Common sleep disorders such as insomnia, sleep apnea, and restless leg syndrome can significantly disrupt hormone balance. Insomnia can lead to inadequate sleep duration and quality, affecting cortisol and melatonin levels. Sleep apnea, characterized by breathing interruptions during sleep, can result in chronic fatigue and hormonal disturbances, particularly affecting women during menopause.

If you suspect a sleep disorder, seek evaluation from a healthcare professional. They can recommend treatments such as cognitive behavioral therapy for insomnia (CBT-I) or continuous positive airway pressure (CPAP) for sleep apnea to restore proper sleep patterns and improve hormonal health.

Techniques for Improving Sleep Hygiene

Improving sleep hygiene involves adopting habits that promote better sleep quality. Start by establishing a consistent sleep schedule, going to bed and waking up at the same time each day, even on weekends. Create a bedtime ritual that signals to your body that it's time to wind down, such as reading a book, taking a warm bath, or practicing relaxation techniques like deep breathing.

Additionally, limit exposure to stimulants such as caffeine and nicotine in the hours leading up to bedtime. Consider incorporating physical activity into your daily routine, as regular exercise can improve sleep quality. Just be mindful to complete workouts earlier in the day, as exercising too close to bedtime may be counterproductive.

The Relationship Between Sleep and Stress Hormones

Sleep and stress hormones, particularly cortisol, have a reciprocal relationship. Chronic stress can lead to elevated cortisol levels, which may inhibit the ability to fall and stay asleep, creating a vicious cycle. High cortisol levels can also disrupt other hormones, leading to symptoms such as weight gain, anxiety, and fatigue.

To manage stress and improve sleep quality, integrate stress-reducing practices into your daily routine. Techniques such as mindfulness meditation, yoga, or journaling can lower cortisol levels and promote relaxation. By prioritizing stress management, you can create a more conducive environment for restorative sleep.

Creating a Bedtime Routine That Promotes Relaxation

A well-structured bedtime routine can signal to your body that it's time to relax and prepare for sleep. Start winding down at least an hour before bedtime by turning off electronic devices and dimming the lights to mimic natural twilight. Engage in calming activities such as reading, gentle stretching, or listening to soothing music to help ease your mind.

Incorporating herbal teas like chamomile or lavender can enhance relaxation and signal your body to prepare for sleep. Establishing this routine consistently will train your body to associate these activities with sleep, making it easier to drift off each night.

The Effects of Blue Light on Sleep Quality

Exposure to blue light from screens can significantly impact sleep quality by suppressing melatonin production. Melatonin is the hormone responsible for regulating sleep-wake cycles, and reduced levels can make it difficult to fall asleep. To mitigate the effects of blue light, limit screen time at least an hour before bed and consider using blue light-blocking glasses.

Additionally, consider using features such as "night mode" on devices, which reduce blue light emission during evening hours. Creating a technology-free zone in your bedroom can further enhance your ability to unwind and prepare for restful sleep.

Natural Sleep Aids to Consider

Natural sleep aids can be effective in promoting better sleep without the side effects associated with pharmaceuticals. Supplements such as melatonin, magnesium, and valerian root are popular choices that can help enhance sleep quality. Always consult with a healthcare professional before starting any new supplements to ensure they're appropriate for your individual needs.

In addition to supplements, consider incorporating herbal teas known for their calming effects, such as chamomile, passionflower, or lemon balm, into your evening routine. These natural aids can support relaxation and help ease you into a restful state.

The Importance of a Comfortable Sleep Environment

A comfortable sleep environment is crucial for quality sleep and hormonal balance. Ensure your bedroom is conducive to rest by keeping the room dark, quiet, and at a comfortable temperature. Invest in a supportive mattress and pillows that cater to your sleeping position to enhance comfort.

Personalize your sleep space with calming colors and textures to create a soothing atmosphere. Consider using blackout curtains to block external light and white noise machines or earplugs to minimize disruptive sounds, promoting a more restful night's sleep.

How to Recognize Signs of Sleep Deprivation

Recognizing the signs of sleep deprivation is vital for addressing sleep issues before they impact your hormonal health. Common signs include persistent fatigue, difficulty concentrating, irritability, and changes in appetite. If you notice these symptoms, it may be time to evaluate your sleep habits and make necessary adjustments.

Keep a sleep journal to track your sleep patterns, noting the hours slept, quality of rest, and any daytime symptoms. This information can help identify trends and patterns that may point to sleep deprivation, allowing you to take proactive steps to improve your sleep quality.

Balancing Sleep with Daily Responsibilities

Finding a balance between sleep and daily responsibilities can be challenging but essential for overall health. Prioritize sleep by scheduling it as you would any important appointment, ensuring you allocate sufficient time for rest. Recognize that adequate sleep will enhance your productivity and energy levels, allowing you to tackle daily tasks more effectively.

To manage your time better, consider implementing time management techniques, such as setting specific goals and breaking tasks into manageable chunks. This approach can help reduce stress and create more opportunities for restorative sleep amid your busy life.

Exploring the Connection Between Sleep and Mood

Sleep significantly influences mood and emotional well-being, with a lack of quality sleep contributing to increased feelings of anxiety and depression. Hormonal fluctuations can also exacerbate these feelings, creating a cycle of poor sleep and emotional distress. Understanding this connection can motivate you to prioritize sleep as a vital component of emotional health.

To enhance your mood through better sleep, focus on creating a positive sleep environment and incorporating relaxation techniques before bed. This will not only improve your sleep quality but can also foster a more positive emotional state during waking hours.

The Long-Term Consequences of Poor Sleep on Hormonal Health

Chronic poor sleep can lead to long-term consequences for hormonal health, including increased risks of conditions like obesity, diabetes, and cardiovascular disease. Hormonal imbalances caused by inadequate sleep can disrupt metabolic processes, leading to weight gain and difficulties in managing stress and emotions.

To mitigate these risks, prioritize sleep as a non-negotiable aspect of your health routine. Regularly assess your sleep patterns and make adjustments as needed to ensure you're getting the quality sleep essential for maintaining hormonal balance and overall health.

CHAPTER 8:

The Impact of Environmental Factors

Understanding Endocrine Disruptors and Their Sources

Endocrine disruptors are chemicals that can interfere with hormonal systems in the body. They are commonly found in everyday products such as plastics, personal care items, pesticides, and even some food packaging. Understanding where these disruptors come from is crucial for minimizing exposure and protecting hormonal balance. Familiarizing yourself with common sources, such as bisphenol A (BPA) in plastics and parabens in cosmetics, can help you make informed choices.

To effectively identify and avoid endocrine disruptors, begin by reading product labels. Look for terms like "fragrance," "parabens," and "phthalates," which are often linked to hormonal interference. Educating yourself about these substances empowers you to choose alternatives that are free from harmful chemicals, ultimately supporting better hormonal health.

How Environmental Toxins Affect Hormonal Balance

Environmental toxins, including heavy metals, pesticides, and industrial chemicals, can significantly impact hormonal balance. These substances may mimic or block hormones, leading to a range of health issues such as irregular menstrual cycles, infertility, and mood disorders. Being aware of the effects of these toxins can help you take proactive measures to safeguard your health.

To mitigate these effects, consider reducing your intake of processed foods, which often contain harmful additives. Incorporating organic produce and grass-fed meats into your diet can lower exposure to pesticides and chemicals. Additionally, advocating for policies that regulate harmful chemicals in your environment can help protect not only your health but also that of your community.

Tips for Reducing Exposure to Harmful Substances

Reducing exposure to harmful substances involves making intentional lifestyle changes. Start by decluttering your home of products that contain known toxins. For instance, replace conventional cleaning supplies with natural alternatives like vinegar and baking soda. Similarly, swap out traditional personal care products for those labeled as organic or free from harmful ingredients.

Another effective strategy is to limit your use of plastic containers, particularly for food storage and microwaving. Opt for glass or stainless steel instead, as they do not leach harmful chemicals. Additionally, practice mindful consumption by choosing products with minimal packaging to reduce waste and exposure to chemicals found in packaging materials.

The Role of Personal Care Products in Hormone Health

Personal care products can be significant sources of endocrine disruptors, affecting hormone health. Many common items like shampoos, lotions, and makeup contain synthetic chemicals that may interfere with hormonal function. Choosing natural or organic personal care products can help mitigate these risks and promote overall wellness.

To transition to safer options, start by evaluating your daily personal care routine. Look for products with simple, recognizable ingredients and avoid those with parabens, phthalates, and sulfates. You can also explore DIY alternatives for common products, such as homemade body scrubs or deodorants, using natural ingredients like coconut oil and essential oils.

Importance of Choosing Organic and Non-Toxic Options

Choosing organic and non-toxic options is essential for maintaining hormonal balance and overall health. Organic foods are grown without synthetic pesticides and fertilizers, reducing exposure to harmful chemicals that can disrupt hormonal function. Likewise, non-toxic household and personal care products are less likely to contain endocrine disruptors.

To incorporate more organic and non-toxic products into your life, start by prioritizing purchases based on the Environmental Working Group's (EWG) "Dirty Dozen" and "Clean Fifteen" lists. Focus on buying organic versions of the most pesticide-laden fruits and vegetables. Additionally, invest in non-toxic cleaning supplies and personal care items to create a healthier living environment.

Exploring the Impact of Plastics on Hormonal Health

Plastics, particularly those containing BPA and phthalates, are known to disrupt hormonal balance. These chemicals can mimic estrogen in the body, potentially leading to reproductive issues and other hormonal imbalances. Understanding the impact of plastics on your health is vital for making informed choices about the products you use.

To reduce plastic exposure, opt for glass or stainless steel containers for food storage and drinking. Avoid heating food in plastic containers, as heat can cause chemicals to leach into your food. Additionally, look for BPA-free labels on plastic products and limit your use of single-use plastics, which contribute to environmental pollution and personal health risks.

The Connection Between Air Quality and Hormones

Air quality plays a crucial role in hormonal health, as exposure to pollutants can disrupt endocrine function. Indoor air pollutants, such as volatile organic compounds (VOCs) from paints and cleaning products, can affect hormone balance and overall well-being. Ensuring good air quality is essential for maintaining hormonal health.

To improve air quality in your home, consider incorporating indoor plants that naturally filter air pollutants. Regularly ventilate your living spaces by opening windows or using air purifiers equipped with HEPA filters. Additionally, choose low-VOC paints and furnishings to reduce harmful emissions in your indoor environment.

How to Create a Safer Home Environment

Creating a safer home environment involves intentional choices that minimize exposure to harmful substances. Start by regularly cleaning your living space with non-toxic cleaning products and ensuring proper ventilation. Use natural materials in your home decor, such as organic cotton and bamboo, which are less likely to emit harmful chemicals.

In addition to cleaning, consider reducing clutter to improve air circulation and minimize dust accumulation. Implement a no-shoes policy indoors to prevent tracking in outside pollutants. By creating a more health-conscious home environment, you can support hormonal balance and enhance overall well-being.

Benefits of Spending Time in Nature for Hormonal Balance

Spending time in nature has numerous benefits for hormonal balance, including stress reduction and improved mood. Nature exposure can lower cortisol levels, a hormone associated with stress, and enhance feelings of relaxation and happiness. Engaging with the natural environment fosters emotional well-being, which is crucial for maintaining hormonal health.

To incorporate more nature into your life, aim for regular outdoor activities such as walking, hiking, or gardening. Even short periods spent in green spaces can have a positive impact on your mental and emotional health. Additionally, consider mindful practices like forest bathing, which involves immersing yourself in nature to promote relaxation and balance.

The Role of Water Quality in Health

Water quality is a critical aspect of overall health, as contaminants can disrupt hormonal balance and impact bodily functions. Pollutants such as heavy metals, chlorine, and pharmaceuticals can enter the water supply and pose health risks. Ensuring access to clean, filtered water is vital for maintaining optimal hormone levels.

To improve water quality, consider investing in a good-quality water filtration system that removes contaminants. Regularly check local water quality reports to stay informed about any potential issues. Additionally, minimize the use of plastic bottles and opt for reusable glass containers to reduce exposure to harmful chemicals often found in plastic.

Educating Yourself About Environmental Health Risks

Education is key to understanding environmental health risks and their impact on hormonal balance. By staying informed about toxins and chemicals in your surroundings, you can make empowered choices to protect your health. Resources such as books, documentaries, and reputable websites provide valuable information on endocrine disruptors and sustainable practices.

Take proactive steps to educate yourself by joining workshops or local community events focused on environmental health. Sharing knowledge with friends and family can also help raise awareness about these issues. Engaging with educational materials can equip you with practical tools to minimize exposure to harmful substances in your daily life.

The Importance of Community Awareness and Advocacy

Community awareness and advocacy play a significant role in promoting environmental health and hormonal balance. By working together, individuals can raise awareness about harmful substances and push for changes in policies that protect public health. Grassroots movements and local initiatives can create lasting impact in addressing environmental risks.

Get involved in your community by participating in local advocacy groups focused on environmental health.

Support initiatives that promote clean air and water, sustainable practices, and reduced exposure to toxins. By collaborating with others, you can amplify your voice and contribute to a healthier environment for everyone.

Strategies for Sustainable Living to Protect Hormones

Sustainable living practices not only benefit the environment but also protect hormonal health. Adopting a lifestyle that prioritizes sustainability involves making conscious choices about consumption, waste, and resource use. Simple actions, such as reducing waste, recycling, and supporting local, organic farmers, can have a positive impact.

Start by implementing small changes in your daily routine, such as using reusable bags, composting kitchen scraps, and opting for public transportation or biking. Additionally, educate yourself on sustainable products and prioritize purchases that align with eco-friendly values.

CHAPTER 9:

Maintaining Hormonal Balance over Time

The Importance of Regular Monitoring of Hormonal Health

Regular monitoring of hormonal health is crucial for identifying imbalances early on, which can lead to significant health issues if left unaddressed. Start by scheduling annual check-ups with a healthcare provider who specializes in hormonal health. Blood tests can measure levels of key hormones like estrogen, progesterone, and testosterone, providing insight into your hormonal status. Tracking symptoms, such as mood swings, fatigue, or changes in menstrual cycles, alongside lab results helps create a comprehensive picture of your health.

To facilitate this process, consider maintaining a health journal where you log symptoms, dietary habits, and lifestyle changes. This documentation not only aids in conversations with your healthcare provider but also helps you notice patterns over time. Make monitoring a part of your routine—setting reminders for appointments and tests can ensure you stay on track with your hormonal health.

Building a Supportive Healthcare Team for Ongoing Care

Creating a supportive healthcare team is essential for comprehensive care in managing hormonal health. Start by identifying a primary care physician who understands hormonal issues, along with specialists such as endocrinologists, nutritionists, or mental health professionals. Establishing clear communication with each member of your team allows for integrated care where everyone is aware of your health goals and treatments.

In addition to professionals, consider involving holistic practitioners such as acupuncturists or herbalists who can offer complementary approaches. Regular meetings or updates with your team can help adjust your care plan as needed. Make sure to ask questions and express concerns openly; an engaged healthcare team is more effective at helping you navigate your hormonal wellness journey.

Understanding the Role of Routine Screenings

Routine screenings play a significant role in maintaining hormonal health by identifying potential issues before they escalate. These screenings can include blood tests, ultrasounds, or mammograms, depending on your age and health history. Familiarize yourself with recommended screening schedules, which can vary based on personal risk factors and family history.

To take advantage of routine screenings, keep a calendar of when tests are due and what your healthcare provider recommends. Approach these appointments with a proactive mindset, using them as opportunities to discuss any changes in your health and to understand what the results mean for your hormonal balance.

Adapting Lifestyle Changes as You Age

As women age, hormonal changes become more pronounced, necessitating adaptations in lifestyle for optimal health. Begin by evaluating your diet, ensuring it includes a variety of whole foods rich in nutrients that support hormonal health, such as leafy greens, lean proteins, and healthy fats. Staying physically active is equally important; aim for at least 150 minutes of moderate exercise each week, including strength training, to support muscle mass and metabolic function.

Additionally, consider incorporating stress management techniques like yoga or meditation into your routine. These practices help mitigate the effects of stress on hormonal balance. Stay informed about changes your body may undergo at different life stages, and be prepared to adjust your lifestyle accordingly to maintain overall wellness.

The Benefits of Continued Education on Hormonal Health

Continued education on hormonal health empowers women to make informed decisions about their well-being. Start by exploring reputable resources such as books, articles, and online courses dedicated to women's health topics. Attending workshops or seminars can also provide valuable insights and the opportunity to engage with experts in the field.

Engaging with educational materials allows you to understand the complexities of hormonal changes and their effects on your body. Consider forming study groups with friends or joining online forums where experiences and knowledge can be shared, making learning a collective journey.

Setting Long-Term Health Goals for Yourself

Setting long-term health goals provides direction and motivation for managing hormonal health. Begin by reflecting on your current state of well-being and identifying areas you'd like to improve, such as weight management, stress reduction, or sleep quality. Use the SMART criteria (Specific, Measurable, Achievable, Relevant, Time-bound) to create clear, attainable goals.

To stay accountable, share your goals with your healthcare team and trusted friends or family members. Regularly reassess your progress and make adjustments as needed; this ensures that your goals remain relevant and motivating as your health journey evolves.

Celebrating Small Wins on Your Wellness Journey

Recognizing and celebrating small wins can significantly enhance your motivation on the wellness journey. Whether it's sticking to a new exercise routine, making healthier food choices, or simply feeling more energetic, acknowledging these achievements reinforces positive behavior. Create a rewards system where you treat yourself to something special, such as a spa day or a new book, to celebrate your progress.

Consider keeping a journal to document your wins, no matter how small. Reflecting on these accomplishments can boost your morale and remind you of how far you've come, fostering a more positive outlook as you navigate the challenges of hormonal health.

Building Resilience to Manage Hormonal Fluctuations

Building resilience is key to managing hormonal fluctuations effectively. Start by developing healthy coping strategies for stress, such as mindfulness practices, regular physical activity, and sufficient sleep. These foundational practices help stabilize mood and energy levels, making it easier to navigate the ups and downs of hormonal changes.

Additionally, cultivate a growth mindset by viewing challenges as opportunities for learning and growth. Surround yourself with supportive people who understand your journey, and don't hesitate to seek professional help if you find it difficult to cope with fluctuations. Remember, resilience is a skill that can be developed over time through consistent practice and self-care.

The Importance of Staying Connected with Support Groups

Staying connected with support groups offers invaluable emotional and practical benefits in managing hormonal health. Start by researching local or online groups focused on women's health, hormonal balance, or specific health conditions. Engaging with others who share similar experiences can provide a sense of community and reduce feelings of isolation.

Participating in these groups allows for sharing strategies, resources, and encouragement. Make it a habit to attend meetings or check in with your group regularly, as these connections can enhance your emotional well-being and provide insights that help you navigate your health journey more effectively.

Encouraging Open Discussions About Hormonal Health

Encouraging open discussions about hormonal health fosters a culture of understanding and support among women. Begin by initiating conversations with friends and family about your experiences and insights. Normalize discussing topics like menstrual cycles, menopause, and hormonal imbalances to break down stigma and promote awareness.

Consider organizing informal gatherings or discussions where women can share their stories and tips related to hormonal health. This openness not only educates others but also builds a supportive network that empowers women to seek help and take charge of their hormonal wellness.

Resources for Ongoing Education and Support

Utilizing various resources for ongoing education and support is essential for managing hormonal health effectively. Start by seeking out reputable websites, such as those from health organizations or medical institutions, which provide evidence-based information on hormonal issues. Online forums and social media groups dedicated to women's health can also be excellent platforms for learning and connecting with others.

Additionally, consider subscribing to newsletters or podcasts focused on hormonal health. These resources can keep you informed about the latest research and trends in women's health, ensuring you stay updated and engaged in your wellness journey.

The Significance of Self-Compassion in the Process

Practicing self-compassion is crucial in navigating the ups and downs of hormonal health. Acknowledge that hormonal changes are a natural part of life, and allow yourself to experience emotions without judgment. Treat yourself with kindness, especially during challenging times, by engaging in self-care activities that bring you joy and relaxation.

Additionally, remind yourself that it's okay to seek help and support when needed. Embracing self-compassion can help reduce stress and promote a positive mindset, making it easier to manage hormonal fluctuations and maintain overall wellness.

Embracing a Lifelong Commitment to Wellness

Embracing a lifelong commitment to wellness is key to maintaining hormonal balance throughout life. Begin by integrating healthy habits into your daily routine, such as balanced nutrition, regular exercise, and mindfulness practices. Consistency is essential; strive to make these habits enjoyable rather than burdensome, fostering a sustainable lifestyle.

As you progress on your wellness journey, stay open to learning and adapting your approach as needed. Regularly revisit your health goals and seek support from your healthcare team and community to ensure you remain on track, fostering a lasting commitment to your well-being.

Common Concerns

What are the signs of hormonal imbalance?

Hormonal imbalance can manifest in various physical and emotional symptoms. Common signs include irregular periods, mood swings, fatigue, weight gain or loss, and changes in sleep patterns. Women may also experience symptoms like hot flashes, breast tenderness, and changes in libido. Recognizing these signs early can help in addressing the underlying issues.

To effectively identify hormonal imbalance, keep a symptom journal. Note any fluctuations in mood, energy levels, or physical changes over time. This record will be invaluable when discussing your symptoms with a healthcare provider, who may suggest tests to assess hormone levels.

How long does it take to restore hormonal balance?

The time required to restore hormonal balance varies from person to person, depending on the severity of the imbalance and the methods used for restoration. Generally, it may take anywhere from a few weeks to several months to see significant changes. Factors such as age, lifestyle, and overall health also influence recovery time.

To expedite the process, maintain consistency with any natural remedies, dietary changes, or supplements recommended by a healthcare professional. Regular follow-ups can help track progress and make necessary adjustments, ensuring you stay on the right path to achieving balance.

Are natural remedies safe to use with medications?

While many natural remedies can be beneficial, it's crucial to consult with a healthcare professional before combining them with medications. Some herbal supplements can interact with prescribed drugs, leading to unwanted side effects or reduced effectiveness. For example, St. John's Wort can interfere with antidepressants, while certain herbs may affect blood sugar levels when taken with diabetes medications.

To ensure safety, always disclose any natural remedies you're considering to your doctor or pharmacist. They can provide guidance on potential interactions and help you determine which combinations are safe and effective for your health needs.

What lifestyle changes have the biggest impact on hormones?

Lifestyle changes can significantly impact hormonal balance, with nutrition and exercise being two of the most influential factors. Adopting a balanced diet rich in whole foods, healthy fats, and lean proteins can provide the nutrients your body needs to produce hormones effectively. Regular physical activity also helps regulate hormone levels by reducing stress and maintaining a healthy weight.

Additionally, prioritize sleep and stress management. Aim for 7-9 hours of quality sleep each night and practice relaxation techniques such as yoga, meditation, or deep breathing exercises. These lifestyle changes can create a positive feedback loop, promoting better hormonal health and overall well-being.

Can hormonal balance improve mental health symptoms?

Restoring hormonal balance can lead to significant improvements in mental health symptoms. Hormones like estrogen, progesterone, and cortisol play critical roles in mood regulation. When these hormones are out of balance, women may experience heightened anxiety, depression, or irritability. By addressing hormonal imbalances, many find relief from these mental health challenges.

To support mental health, consider incorporating lifestyle changes that promote hormonal balance, such as regular exercise, a healthy diet, and adequate sleep. In some cases, working with a healthcare professional who specializes in hormonal health can provide tailored strategies and support to improve both hormonal and mental well-being.

FAQs

What should I do if I suspect a hormonal imbalance?

If you suspect a hormonal imbalance, the first step is to consult a healthcare professional who can conduct appropriate tests. Blood tests or hormone panels can help identify specific hormonal deficiencies or excesses. This is crucial for understanding your unique situation and determining the best course of action.

Once you have your test results, discuss them with your healthcare provider to develop a personalized plan. This might include lifestyle modifications, dietary changes, or medication options. Always seek professional guidance to ensure you're addressing the root cause of your hormonal issues effectively.

How can I track my hormonal health?

Tracking your hormonal health is essential for identifying patterns and triggers. Start by keeping a journal to document your symptoms, menstrual cycles, mood changes, and lifestyle factors such as diet, sleep, and stress levels. This will give you a clearer picture of your hormonal fluctuations over time.

You can also use mobile apps specifically designed for tracking hormonal health. These apps often allow you to record symptoms and cycle information, providing visual data to share with your healthcare provider. This tracking will empower you to take control of your health and facilitate informed discussions with your doctor.

What is the best diet for hormonal balance?

A balanced diet plays a significant role in maintaining hormonal balance. Focus on whole foods, incorporating healthy fats like avocados, nuts, and olive oil, as they support hormone production. Include plenty of fruits and vegetables, particularly those high in fiber, which helps regulate estrogen levels.

Additionally, reduce your intake of processed foods, sugar, and caffeine, as these can exacerbate hormonal imbalances. Planning meals that prioritize nutrient-dense options will not only support your hormones but also promote overall health. Consider consulting with a nutritionist to tailor your diet to your specific needs.

Are there specific exercises that help with hormonal balance?

Exercise is a powerful tool for managing hormonal health. Strength training is particularly beneficial, as it helps build muscle mass, which can enhance metabolism and improve insulin sensitivity. Aim for at least two to three sessions per week, focusing on major muscle groups.

Incorporate yoga and moderate aerobic activities into your routine, as they can help reduce stress levels and improve mood. Activities like walking, cycling, or swimming can also support hormonal balance by promoting overall fitness and well-being. Establish a consistent exercise schedule that feels enjoyable and sustainable for you.

When should I seek medical advice for hormonal issues?

It's important to seek medical advice for hormonal issues if you experience persistent symptoms such as extreme fatigue, irregular periods, mood swings, or weight changes. These signs may indicate an underlying hormonal imbalance that requires professional intervention.

If your symptoms significantly impact your daily life or worsen over time, don't hesitate to consult a healthcare provider. Early intervention can prevent complications and help you find effective solutions tailored to your specific hormonal health needs. Prioritize your well-being and take proactive steps towards achieving balance.

Conclusion

Achieving Hormonal Balance: A Holistic Journey

Achieving hormonal balance is a journey that requires a holistic approach, addressing the body, mind, and spirit. Start by assessing your current lifestyle, including diet, exercise, stress management, and sleep patterns. Keeping a journal can help identify triggers and patterns affecting your hormones. Once you understand these factors, implement gradual changes such as incorporating regular physical activity, practicing mindfulness techniques, and prioritizing restorative sleep.

Additionally, consider seeking guidance from health professionals who can provide personalized recommendations based on your individual needs. Integrating holistic practices such as yoga, meditation, and herbal remedies can further support hormonal balance. Remember, this journey is not a quick fix; it's about cultivating sustainable habits that promote long-term well-being.

Understanding the Interplay of Lifestyle, Nutrition, and Self-Care

Understanding the interplay of lifestyle, nutrition, and self-care is crucial for taking charge of your hormonal health. Start with nutrition by focusing on whole foods rich in nutrients that support hormone regulation, such as leafy greens, healthy fats, and lean proteins. Reduce processed foods and sugar intake, as these can cause hormonal imbalances. Keeping a balanced diet helps maintain stable blood sugar levels, which is vital for hormonal health.

Incorporate self-care practices into your daily routine to reduce stress and enhance emotional well-being. Techniques such as deep breathing exercises, regular physical activity, and engaging in hobbies you enjoy can significantly impact hormonal balance. By paying attention to both nutrition and self-care, you can create a supportive environment for your hormones to thrive.

The Importance of Ongoing Education

Ongoing education is essential for maintaining hormonal balance and enhancing overall well-being. Start by researching reliable sources, such as books, podcasts, and reputable health websites, to deepen your understanding of hormonal health. Join workshops or support groups to share experiences and learn from others facing similar challenges. Staying informed about the latest research can empower you to make educated decisions about your health.

Additionally, consider working with health practitioners who specialize in hormonal balance, such as nutritionists or integrative health coaches. They can provide tailored advice and help you navigate your journey. Continuous learning and support will reinforce your commitment to achieving and maintaining hormonal balance, ultimately leading to improved wellness.

Incorporating Regular Exercise

Incorporating regular exercise is a fundamental aspect of achieving hormonal balance. Aim for at least 150 minutes of moderate aerobic activity per week, such as brisk walking, cycling, or swimming. Exercise helps regulate insulin levels, improve mood, and reduce stress, all of which are vital for hormonal health. Consider adding strength training exercises to your routine two to three times a week, as this can boost metabolism and promote muscle growth.

Finding activities you enjoy will make it easier to stay consistent. Whether it's dancing, hiking, or participating in group classes, making exercise fun can enhance your motivation. Additionally, listen to your body and adjust your workout intensity according to your energy levels, ensuring you maintain a sustainable exercise routine.

Prioritizing Nutrition for Hormonal Health

Prioritizing nutrition is crucial for maintaining hormonal health. Focus on incorporating a variety of nutrient-dense foods, such as fruits, vegetables, whole grains, lean proteins, and healthy fats into your meals. Foods rich in omega-3 fatty acids, like fatty fish and walnuts, can help reduce inflammation and support hormonal function. Consider keeping a food diary to track what you eat and identify any foods that may trigger hormonal imbalances.

Moreover, staying hydrated is essential for overall health and can aid in hormone regulation. Aim to drink plenty of water throughout the day and consider herbal teas that can provide additional benefits, such as peppermint or chamomile. By making informed dietary choices and staying hydrated, you can support your body's natural hormonal balance.

Managing Stress Effectively

Managing stress effectively is vital for hormonal balance. Start by identifying stressors in your life and implementing strategies to address them. This might include setting boundaries, practicing time management, or seeking support from friends and family. Incorporating relaxation techniques, such as deep breathing, progressive muscle relaxation, or mindfulness meditation, can also significantly reduce stress levels.

Creating a routine that includes regular breaks for self-care is essential. Engage in activities that bring you joy, such as reading, gardening, or spending time with loved ones. By actively managing stress and creating a balanced lifestyle, you can mitigate its negative impact on your hormones and improve your overall well-being.

Emphasizing Quality Sleep

Emphasizing quality sleep is critical for maintaining hormonal balance. Establish a consistent sleep schedule by going to bed and waking up at the same time each day, even on weekends. Create a calming bedtime routine that may include activities like reading, taking a warm bath, or practicing relaxation techniques to signal to your body that it's time to wind down.

Consider your sleep environment: ensure it's dark, quiet, and at a comfortable temperature. Limit screen time before bed, as blue light from devices can interfere with melatonin production. By prioritizing sleep hygiene and making adjustments to your routine, you can significantly enhance the quality of your sleep, which is essential for hormone regulation.

Exploring Herbal Remedies

Exploring herbal remedies can be a beneficial way to support hormonal balance. Herbs like chaste tree berry (Vitex), ashwagandha, and maca root have been traditionally used to help regulate hormones and alleviate symptoms associated with hormonal imbalances. Start by researching these herbs and their potential benefits, and consider incorporating them into your routine in consultation with a healthcare provider.

When using herbal remedies, it's essential to follow dosage guidelines and monitor how your body responds. Keep a journal to track any changes in your symptoms and overall well-being. By taking a cautious and informed approach, you can effectively utilize herbal remedies as part of your holistic strategy for achieving hormonal balance.

Building a Support Network

Building a support network is crucial for maintaining hormonal balance. Surround yourself with friends, family, or community groups that understand your journey and can provide encouragement. Consider joining online forums or local support groups where you can share experiences, challenges, and successes related to hormonal health.

Additionally, don't hesitate to seek professional help from practitioners such as nutritionists, therapists, or holistic health coaches. Having a supportive community can motivate you to stay committed to your health goals and offer valuable insights and resources. By fostering connections with others, you can enhance your understanding and commitment to achieving hormonal balance.

Tracking Your Progress

Tracking your progress is an essential step in managing hormonal health. Use a journal or digital app to log your daily habits, including nutrition, exercise, sleep patterns, and mood changes. Regularly review this information to identify patterns and areas where adjustments may be needed. This practice will help you stay accountable and provide insights into what strategies are most effective for you.

Set realistic goals for your hormonal health journey, and celebrate small achievements along the way. Whether it's trying a new healthy recipe, completing a week of consistent exercise, or improving sleep quality, recognizing these milestones can boost your motivation. By actively tracking your progress, you'll gain a clearer understanding of your body's needs and how to best support your hormonal balance.

Practicing Mindfulness and Meditation

Practicing mindfulness and meditation can significantly enhance your journey toward hormonal balance. Begin by setting aside a few minutes each day to focus on your breath and clear your mind. Techniques like guided meditation, body scans, or mindfulness-based stress reduction can help cultivate awareness and reduce stress, which is vital for hormonal health.

Incorporate mindfulness into your daily activities by being fully present in the moment, whether you're eating, exercising, or spending time with loved ones. By regularly practicing mindfulness and meditation, you can develop a deeper connection with your body and emotions, fostering a sense of calm that supports hormonal balance and overall well-being.

Seeking Professional Guidance

Seeking professional guidance is an important aspect of achieving and maintaining hormonal balance. Consider consulting with a healthcare provider who specializes in women's health or hormonal issues. They can conduct assessments, recommend appropriate tests, and develop a personalized plan to address your specific hormonal needs.

Be proactive in communicating your symptoms and concerns during your appointments. This collaboration will help your healthcare provider tailor their approach to your unique situation. Additionally, exploring various professionals, such as nutritionists, therapists, or holistic health practitioners, can provide you with diverse perspectives and strategies to support your hormonal health journey.